Guests

ADVICE FOR PARENTS (WE NEED IT)

WISHES FOR THE MINI POOP MACHINE

SLEEP (OR TRANQUILIZER) SUGGESTIONS

YOU'RE KINDA GLA̲̲̲̲̲̲̲̲̲̲̲̲̲̲̲̲̲̲̲̲̲GHT?

WILL YOU TAKE THIS CHILD IF WE CAN'T COPE?

Guests

ADVICE FOR PARENTS (WE NEED IT)

_____

_____

_____

WISHES FOR THE MINI POOP MACHINE

_____

_____

_____

SLEEP (OR TRANQUILIZER) SUGGESTIONS

_____

YOU'RE KINDA GLAD IT'S NOT YOU, RIGHT?

_____

WILL YOU TAKE THIS CHILD IF WE CAN'T COPE?

_____

Guests

ADVICE FOR PARENTS (WE NEED IT)

_____

_____

_____

WISHES FOR THE MINI POOP MACHINE

_____

_____

_____

SLEEP (OR TRANQUILIZER) SUGGESTIONS

_____

YOU'RE KINDA GLAD IT'S NOT YOU, RIGHT?

_____

WILL YOU TAKE THIS CHILD IF WE CAN'T COPE?

_____

Guests

ADVICE FOR PARENTS (WE NEED IT)

WISHES FOR THE MINI POOP MACHINE

SLEEP (OR TRANQUILIZER) SUGGESTIONS

YOU'RE KINDA GLAD IT'S NOT YOU, RIGHT?

WILL YOU TAKE THIS CHILD IF WE CAN'T COPE?

Guests

_____

ADVICE FOR PARENTS (WE NEED IT)

_____

_____

_____

WISHES FOR THE MINI POOP MACHINE

_____

_____

_____

SLEEP (OR TRANQUILIZER) SUGGESTIONS

_____

YOU'RE KINDA GLAD IT'S NOT YOU, RIGHT?

_____

WILL YOU TAKE THIS CHILD IF WE CAN'T COPE?

_____

Guests

___

ADVICE FOR PARENTS (WE NEED IT)

___

___

___

WISHES FOR THE MINI POOP MACHINE

___

___

___

SLEEP (OR TRANQUILIZER) SUGGESTIONS

___

YOU'RE KINDA GLAD IT'S NOT YOU, RIGHT?

___

WILL YOU TAKE THIS CHILD IF WE CAN'T COPE?

___

Guests

ADVICE FOR PARENTS (WE NEED IT)

WISHES FOR THE MINI POOP MACHINE

SLEEP (OR TRANQUILIZER) SUGGESTIONS

YOU'RE KINDA GLAD IT'S NOT YOU, RIGHT?

WILL YOU TAKE THIS CHILD IF WE CAN'T COPE?

Guests

ADVICE FOR PARENTS (WE NEED IT)

_____

_____

_____

WISHES FOR THE MINI POOP MACHINE

_____

_____

_____

SLEEP (OR TRANQUILIZER) SUGGESTIONS

_____

YOU'RE KINDA GLAD IT'S NOT YOU, RIGHT?

_____

WILL YOU TAKE THIS CHILD IF WE CAN'T COPE?

_____

Guests

_____

ADVICE FOR PARENTS (WE NEED IT)

_____

_____

_____

WISHES FOR THE MINI POOP MACHINE

_____

_____

_____

SLEEP (OR TRANQUILIZER) SUGGESTIONS

_____

YOU'RE KINDA GLAD IT'S NOT YOU, RIGHT?

_____

WILL YOU TAKE THIS CHILD IF WE CAN'T COPE?

_____

Guests

ADVICE FOR PARENTS (WE NEED IT)

_____

_____

_____

WISHES FOR THE MINI POOP MACHINE

_____

_____

_____

SLEEP (OR TRANQUILIZER) SUGGESTIONS

_____

YOU'RE KINDA GLAD IT'S NOT YOU, RIGHT?

_____

WILL YOU TAKE THIS CHILD IF WE CAN'T COPE?

_____

Guests

_____

ADVICE FOR PARENTS (WE NEED IT)

_____

_____

_____

WISHES FOR THE MINI POOP MACHINE

_____

_____

_____

SLEEP (OR TRANQUILIZER) SUGGESTIONS

_____

YOU'RE KINDA GLAD IT'S NOT YOU, RIGHT?

_____

WILL YOU TAKE THIS CHILD IF WE CAN'T COPE?

_____

Guests

___

ADVICE FOR PARENTS (WE NEED IT)

___

___

___

WISHES FOR THE MINI POOP MACHINE

___

___

___

SLEEP (OR TRANQUILIZER) SUGGESTIONS

___

YOU'RE KINDA GLAD IT'S NOT YOU, RIGHT?

___

WILL YOU TAKE THIS CHILD IF WE CAN'T COPE?

___

Guests

_____

ADVICE FOR PARENTS (WE NEED IT)

_____

_____

_____

WISHES FOR THE MINI POOP MACHINE

_____

_____

_____

SLEEP (OR TRANQUILIZER) SUGGESTIONS

_____

YOU'RE KINDA GLAD IT'S NOT YOU, RIGHT?

_____

WILL YOU TAKE THIS CHILD IF WE CAN'T COPE?

_____

Guests

ADVICE FOR PARENTS (WE NEED IT)

_____

_____

_____

WISHES FOR THE MINI POOP MACHINE

_____

_____

_____

SLEEP (OR TRANQUILIZER) SUGGESTIONS

_____

YOU'RE KINDA GLAD IT'S NOT YOU, RIGHT?

_____

WILL YOU TAKE THIS CHILD IF WE CAN'T COPE?

_____

Guests

___

ADVICE FOR PARENTS (WE NEED IT)

___

___

___

WISHES FOR THE MINI POOP MACHINE

___

___

___

SLEEP (OR TRANQUILIZER) SUGGESTIONS

___

YOU'RE KINDA GLAD IT'S NOT YOU, RIGHT?

___

WILL YOU TAKE THIS CHILD IF WE CAN'T COPE?

___

Guests

ADVICE FOR PARENTS (WE NEED IT)

_____

_____

_____

WISHES FOR THE MINI POOP MACHINE

_____

_____

_____

SLEEP (OR TRANQUILIZER) SUGGESTIONS

_____

YOU'RE KINDA GLAD IT'S NOT YOU, RIGHT?

_____

WILL YOU TAKE THIS CHILD IF WE CAN'T COPE?

_____

Guests

_____

ADVICE FOR PARENTS (WE NEED IT)

_____

_____

_____

WISHES FOR THE MINI POOP MACHINE

_____

_____

_____

SLEEP (OR TRANQUILIZER) SUGGESTIONS

_____

YOU'RE KINDA GLAD IT'S NOT YOU, RIGHT?

_____

WILL YOU TAKE THIS CHILD IF WE CAN'T COPE?

_____

Guests

_____

ADVICE FOR PARENTS (WE NEED IT)

_____

_____

_____

WISHES FOR THE MINI POOP MACHINE

_____

_____

_____

SLEEP (OR TRANQUILIZER) SUGGESTIONS

_____

YOU'RE KINDA GLAD IT'S NOT YOU, RIGHT?

_____

WILL YOU TAKE THIS CHILD IF WE CAN'T COPE?

_____

Guests

ADVICE FOR PARENTS (WE NEED IT)

WISHES FOR THE MINI POOP MACHINE

SLEEP (OR TRANQUILIZER) SUGGESTIONS

YOU'RE KINDA GLAD IT'S NOT YOU, RIGHT?

WILL YOU TAKE THIS CHILD IF WE CAN'T COPE?

Guests

ADVICE FOR PARENTS (WE NEED IT)

_____

_____

_____

WISHES FOR THE MINI POOP MACHINE

_____

_____

_____

SLEEP (OR TRANQUILIZER) SUGGESTIONS

_____

YOU'RE KINDA GLAD IT'S NOT YOU, RIGHT?

_____

WILL YOU TAKE THIS CHILD IF WE CAN'T COPE?

_____

Guests

_____

ADVICE FOR PARENTS (WE NEED IT)

_____

_____

_____

WISHES FOR THE MINI POOP MACHINE

_____

_____

_____

SLEEP (OR TRANQUILIZER) SUGGESTIONS

_____

YOU'RE KINDA GLAD IT'S NOT YOU, RIGHT?

_____

WILL YOU TAKE THIS CHILD IF WE CAN'T COPE?

_____

Guests

ADVICE FOR PARENTS (WE NEED IT)

_____

_____

_____

WISHES FOR THE MINI POOP MACHINE

_____

_____

_____

SLEEP (OR TRANQUILIZER) SUGGESTIONS

_____

YOU'RE KINDA GLAD IT'S NOT YOU, RIGHT?

_____

WILL YOU TAKE THIS CHILD IF WE CAN'T COPE?

_____

Guests

_____

ADVICE FOR PARENTS (WE NEED IT)

_____

_____

_____

WISHES FOR THE MINI POOP MACHINE

_____

_____

_____

SLEEP (OR TRANQUILIZER) SUGGESTIONS

_____

YOU'RE KINDA GLAD IT'S NOT YOU, RIGHT?

_____

WILL YOU TAKE THIS CHILD IF WE CAN'T COPE?

_____

Guests

ADVICE FOR PARENTS (WE NEED IT)

WISHES FOR THE MINI POOP MACHINE

SLEEP (OR TRANQUILIZER) SUGGESTIONS

YOU'RE KINDA GLAD IT'S NOT YOU, RIGHT?

WILL YOU TAKE THIS CHILD IF WE CAN'T COPE?

Guests

_____

ADVICE FOR PARENTS (WE NEED IT)

_____

_____

_____

WISHES FOR THE MINI POOP MACHINE

_____

_____

_____

SLEEP (OR TRANQUILIZER) SUGGESTIONS

_____

YOU'RE KINDA GLAD IT'S NOT YOU, RIGHT?

_____

WILL YOU TAKE THIS CHILD IF WE CAN'T COPE?

_____

Guests

ADVICE FOR PARENTS (WE NEED IT)

_____

_____

_____

WISHES FOR THE MINI POOP MACHINE

_____

_____

_____

SLEEP (OR TRANQUILIZER) SUGGESTIONS

_____

YOU'RE KINDA GLAD IT'S NOT YOU, RIGHT?

_____

WILL YOU TAKE THIS CHILD IF WE CAN'T COPE?

_____

Guests

_____

ADVICE FOR PARENTS (WE NEED IT)

_____

_____

_____

WISHES FOR THE MINI POOP MACHINE

_____

_____

_____

SLEEP (OR TRANQUILIZER) SUGGESTIONS

_____

YOU'RE KINDA GLAD IT'S NOT YOU, RIGHT?

_____

WILL YOU TAKE THIS CHILD IF WE CAN'T COPE?

_____

Guests

ADVICE FOR PARENTS (WE NEED IT)

_____

_____

_____

WISHES FOR THE MINI POOP MACHINE

_____

_____

_____

SLEEP (OR TRANQUILIZER) SUGGESTIONS

_____

YOU'RE KINDA GLAD IT'S NOT YOU, RIGHT?

_____

WILL YOU TAKE THIS CHILD IF WE CAN'T COPE?

_____

Guests

_____

ADVICE FOR PARENTS (WE NEED IT)

_____

_____

_____

WISHES FOR THE MINI POOP MACHINE

_____

_____

_____

SLEEP (OR TRANQUILIZER) SUGGESTIONS

_____

YOU'RE KINDA GLAD IT'S NOT YOU, RIGHT?

_____

WILL YOU TAKE THIS CHILD IF WE CAN'T COPE?

_____

Guests

ADVICE FOR PARENTS (WE NEED IT)

WISHES FOR THE MINI POOP MACHINE

SLEEP (OR TRANQUILIZER) SUGGESTIONS

YOU'RE KINDA GLAD IT'S NOT YOU, RIGHT?

WILL YOU TAKE THIS CHILD IF WE CAN'T COPE?

Guests

_____

ADVICE FOR PARENTS (WE NEED IT)

_____

_____

_____

WISHES FOR THE MINI POOP MACHINE

_____

_____

_____

SLEEP (OR TRANQUILIZER) SUGGESTIONS

_____

YOU'RE KINDA GLAD IT'S NOT YOU, RIGHT?

_____

WILL YOU TAKE THIS CHILD IF WE CAN'T COPE?

_____

Guests

ADVICE FOR PARENTS (WE NEED IT)

_____

_____

_____

WISHES FOR THE MINI POOP MACHINE

_____

_____

_____

SLEEP (OR TRANQUILIZER) SUGGESTIONS

_____

YOU'RE KINDA GLAD IT'S NOT YOU, RIGHT?

_____

WILL YOU TAKE THIS CHILD IF WE CAN'T COPE?

_____

Guests

_____

ADVICE FOR PARENTS (WE NEED IT)

_____

_____

_____

WISHES FOR THE MINI POOP MACHINE

_____

_____

_____

SLEEP (OR TRANQUILIZER) SUGGESTIONS

_____

YOU'RE KINDA GLAD IT'S NOT YOU, RIGHT?

_____

WILL YOU TAKE THIS CHILD IF WE CAN'T COPE?

_____

Guests

ADVICE FOR PARENTS (WE NEED IT)

_____

_____

_____

WISHES FOR THE MINI POOP MACHINE

_____

_____

_____

SLEEP (OR TRANQUILIZER) SUGGESTIONS

_____

YOU'RE KINDA GLAD IT'S NOT YOU, RIGHT?

_____

WILL YOU TAKE THIS CHILD IF WE CAN'T COPE?

_____

Guests

_____

ADVICE FOR PARENTS (WE NEED IT)

_____

_____

_____

WISHES FOR THE MINI POOP MACHINE

_____

_____

_____

SLEEP (OR TRANQUILIZER) SUGGESTIONS

_____

YOU'RE KINDA GLAD IT'S NOT YOU, RIGHT?

_____

WILL YOU TAKE THIS CHILD IF WE CAN'T COPE?

_____

Guests

ADVICE FOR PARENTS (WE NEED IT)

WISHES FOR THE MINI POOP MACHINE

SLEEP (OR TRANQUILIZER) SUGGESTIONS

YOU'RE KINDA GLAD IT'S NOT YOU, RIGHT?

WILL YOU TAKE THIS CHILD IF WE CAN'T COPE?

Guests

_____

ADVICE FOR PARENTS (WE NEED IT)

_____

_____

_____

WISHES FOR THE MINI POOP MACHINE

_____

_____

_____

SLEEP (OR TRANQUILIZER) SUGGESTIONS

_____

YOU'RE KINDA GLAD IT'S NOT YOU, RIGHT?

_____

WILL YOU TAKE THIS CHILD IF WE CAN'T COPE?

_____

Guests

_____

ADVICE FOR PARENTS (WE NEED IT)

_____

_____

_____

WISHES FOR THE MINI POOP MACHINE

_____

_____

_____

SLEEP (OR TRANQUILIZER) SUGGESTIONS

_____

YOU'RE KINDA GLAD IT'S NOT YOU, RIGHT?

_____

WILL YOU TAKE THIS CHILD IF WE CAN'T COPE?

_____

Guests

ADVICE FOR PARENTS (WE NEED IT)

_____

_____

_____

WISHES FOR THE MINI POOP MACHINE

_____

_____

_____

SLEEP (OR TRANQUILIZER) SUGGESTIONS

_____

YOU'RE KINDA GLAD IT'S NOT YOU, RIGHT?

_____

WILL YOU TAKE THIS CHILD IF WE CAN'T COPE?

_____

Guests

ADVICE FOR PARENTS (WE NEED IT)

_____

_____

_____

WISHES FOR THE MINI POOP MACHINE

_____

_____

_____

SLEEP (OR TRANQUILIZER) SUGGESTIONS

_____

YOU'RE KINDA GLAD IT'S NOT YOU, RIGHT?

_____

WILL YOU TAKE THIS CHILD IF WE CAN'T COPE?

_____

Guests

_____

ADVICE FOR PARENTS (WE NEED IT)

_____

_____

_____

WISHES FOR THE MINI POOP MACHINE

_____

_____

_____

SLEEP (OR TRANQUILIZER) SUGGESTIONS

_____

YOU'RE KINDA GLAD IT'S NOT YOU, RIGHT?

_____

WILL YOU TAKE THIS CHILD IF WE CAN'T COPE?

_____

Guests

_____

ADVICE FOR PARENTS (WE NEED IT)

_____

_____

_____

WISHES FOR THE MINI POOP MACHINE

_____

_____

_____

SLEEP (OR TRANQUILIZER) SUGGESTIONS

_____

YOU'RE KINDA GLAD IT'S NOT YOU, RIGHT?

_____

WILL YOU TAKE THIS CHILD IF WE CAN'T COPE?

_____

Guests

_____

ADVICE FOR PARENTS (WE NEED IT)

_____

_____

WISHES FOR THE MINI POOP MACHINE

_____

_____

SLEEP (OR TRANQUILIZER) SUGGESTIONS

_____

YOU'RE KINDA GLAD IT'S NOT YOU, RIGHT?

_____

WILL YOU TAKE THIS CHILD IF WE CAN'T COPE?

_____

Guests

ADVICE FOR PARENTS (WE NEED IT)

_____

_____

_____

WISHES FOR THE MINI POOP MACHINE

_____

_____

_____

SLEEP (OR TRANQUILIZER) SUGGESTIONS

_____

YOU'RE KINDA GLAD IT'S NOT YOU, RIGHT?

_____

WILL YOU TAKE THIS CHILD IF WE CAN'T COPE?

_____

Guests

ADVICE FOR PARENTS (WE NEED IT)

WISHES FOR THE MINI POOP MACHINE

SLEEP (OR TRANQUILIZER) SUGGESTIONS

YOU'RE KINDA GLAD IT'S NOT YOU, RIGHT?

WILL YOU TAKE THIS CHILD IF WE CAN'T COPE?

Guests

ADVICE FOR PARENTS (WE NEED IT)

_____

_____

_____

WISHES FOR THE MINI POOP MACHINE

_____

_____

_____

SLEEP (OR TRANQUILIZER) SUGGESTIONS

_____

YOU'RE KINDA GLAD IT'S NOT YOU, RIGHT?

_____

WILL YOU TAKE THIS CHILD IF WE CAN'T COPE?

_____

Guests

_____

ADVICE FOR PARENTS (WE NEED IT)

_____

_____

_____

WISHES FOR THE MINI POOP MACHINE

_____

_____

_____

SLEEP (OR TRANQUILIZER) SUGGESTIONS

_____

YOU'RE KINDA GLAD IT'S NOT YOU, RIGHT?

_____

WILL YOU TAKE THIS CHILD IF WE CAN'T COPE?

_____

Guests

ADVICE FOR PARENTS (WE NEED IT)

_____

_____

_____

WISHES FOR THE MINI POOP MACHINE

_____

_____

_____

SLEEP (OR TRANQUILIZER) SUGGESTIONS

_____

YOU'RE KINDA GLAD IT'S NOT YOU, RIGHT?

_____

WILL YOU TAKE THIS CHILD IF WE CAN'T COPE?

_____

Guests

_____

ADVICE FOR PARENTS (WE NEED IT)

_____

_____

WISHES FOR THE MINI POOP MACHINE

_____

_____

SLEEP (OR TRANQUILIZER) SUGGESTIONS

_____

YOU'RE KINDA GLAD IT'S NOT YOU, RIGHT?

_____

WILL YOU TAKE THIS CHILD IF WE CAN'T COPE?

_____

Guests

ADVICE FOR PARENTS (WE NEED IT)

WISHES FOR THE MINI POOP MACHINE

SLEEP (OR TRANQUILIZER) SUGGESTIONS

YOU'RE KINDA GLAD IT'S NOT YOU, RIGHT?

WILL YOU TAKE THIS CHILD IF WE CAN'T COPE?

Guests

_____

ADVICE FOR PARENTS (WE NEED IT)

_____

_____

WISHES FOR THE MINI POOP MACHINE

_____

_____

SLEEP (OR TRANQUILIZER) SUGGESTIONS

_____

YOU'RE KINDA GLAD IT'S NOT YOU, RIGHT?

_____

WILL YOU TAKE THIS CHILD IF WE CAN'T COPE?

_____

Guests

ADVICE FOR PARENTS (WE NEED IT)

_____

_____

_____

WISHES FOR THE MINI POOP MACHINE

_____

_____

_____

SLEEP (OR TRANQUILIZER) SUGGESTIONS

_____

YOU'RE KINDA GLAD IT'S NOT YOU, RIGHT?

_____

WILL YOU TAKE THIS CHILD IF WE CAN'T COPE?

_____

Guests

_____

ADVICE FOR PARENTS (WE NEED IT)

_____

_____

_____

WISHES FOR THE MINI POOP MACHINE

_____

_____

_____

SLEEP (OR TRANQUILIZER) SUGGESTIONS

_____

YOU'RE KINDA GLAD IT'S NOT YOU, RIGHT?

_____

WILL YOU TAKE THIS CHILD IF WE CAN'T COPE?

_____

Guests

ADVICE FOR PARENTS (WE NEED IT)

_____

_____

_____

WISHES FOR THE MINI POOP MACHINE

_____

_____

_____

SLEEP (OR TRANQUILIZER) SUGGESTIONS

_____

YOU'RE KINDA GLAD IT'S NOT YOU, RIGHT?

_____

WILL YOU TAKE THIS CHILD IF WE CAN'T COPE?

_____

Guests

_____

ADVICE FOR PARENTS (WE NEED IT)

_____

_____

_____

WISHES FOR THE MINI POOP MACHINE

_____

_____

_____

SLEEP (OR TRANQUILIZER) SUGGESTIONS

_____

YOU'RE KINDA GLAD IT'S NOT YOU, RIGHT?

_____

WILL YOU TAKE THIS CHILD IF WE CAN'T COPE?

_____

Guests

ADVICE FOR PARENTS (WE NEED IT)

_____

_____

_____

WISHES FOR THE MINI POOP MACHINE

_____

_____

_____

SLEEP (OR TRANQUILIZER) SUGGESTIONS

_____

YOU'RE KINDA GLAD IT'S NOT YOU, RIGHT?

_____

WILL YOU TAKE THIS CHILD IF WE CAN'T COPE?

_____

Guests

ADVICE FOR PARENTS (WE NEED IT)

WISHES FOR THE MINI POOP MACHINE

SLEEP (OR TRANQUILIZER) SUGGESTIONS

YOU'RE KINDA GLAD IT'S NOT YOU, RIGHT?

WILL YOU TAKE THIS CHILD IF WE CAN'T COPE?

Guests

ADVICE FOR PARENTS (WE NEED IT)

_____

_____

_____

WISHES FOR THE MINI POOP MACHINE

_____

_____

_____

SLEEP (OR TRANQUILIZER) SUGGESTIONS

_____

YOU'RE KINDA GLAD IT'S NOT YOU, RIGHT?

_____

WILL YOU TAKE THIS CHILD IF WE CAN'T COPE?

_____

Guests

_____

ADVICE FOR PARENTS (WE NEED IT)

_____

_____

_____

WISHES FOR THE MINI POOP MACHINE

_____

_____

_____

SLEEP (OR TRANQUILIZER) SUGGESTIONS

_____

YOU'RE KINDA GLAD IT'S NOT YOU, RIGHT?

_____

WILL YOU TAKE THIS CHILD IF WE CAN'T COPE?

_____

Guests

ADVICE FOR PARENTS (WE NEED IT)

WISHES FOR THE MINI POOP MACHINE

SLEEP (OR TRANQUILIZER) SUGGESTIONS

YOU'RE KINDA GLAD IT'S NOT YOU, RIGHT?

WILL YOU TAKE THIS CHILD IF WE CAN'T COPE?

Guests

_____

ADVICE FOR PARENTS (WE NEED IT)

_____

_____

_____

WISHES FOR THE MINI POOP MACHINE

_____

_____

_____

SLEEP (OR TRANQUILIZER) SUGGESTIONS

_____

YOU'RE KINDA GLAD IT'S NOT YOU, RIGHT?

_____

WILL YOU TAKE THIS CHILD IF WE CAN'T COPE?

_____

Guests

ADVICE FOR PARENTS (WE NEED IT)

_____

_____

_____

WISHES FOR THE MINI POOP MACHINE

_____

_____

_____

SLEEP (OR TRANQUILIZER) SUGGESTIONS

_____

YOU'RE KINDA GLAD IT'S NOT YOU, RIGHT?

_____

WILL YOU TAKE THIS CHILD IF WE CAN'T COPE?

_____

Guests

_____

ADVICE FOR PARENTS (WE NEED IT)

_____

_____

_____

WISHES FOR THE MINI POOP MACHINE

_____

_____

_____

SLEEP (OR TRANQUILIZER) SUGGESTIONS

_____

YOU'RE KINDA GLAD IT'S NOT YOU, RIGHT?

_____

WILL YOU TAKE THIS CHILD IF WE CAN'T COPE?

_____

Guests

ADVICE FOR PARENTS (WE NEED IT)

_____

_____

_____

WISHES FOR THE MINI POOP MACHINE

_____

_____

_____

SLEEP (OR TRANQUILIZER) SUGGESTIONS

_____

YOU'RE KINDA GLAD IT'S NOT YOU, RIGHT?

_____

WILL YOU TAKE THIS CHILD IF WE CAN'T COPE?

_____

Guests

_____

ADVICE FOR PARENTS (WE NEED IT)

_____

_____

_____

WISHES FOR THE MINI POOP MACHINE

_____

_____

_____

SLEEP (OR TRANQUILIZER) SUGGESTIONS

_____

YOU'RE KINDA GLAD IT'S NOT YOU, RIGHT?

_____

WILL YOU TAKE THIS CHILD IF WE CAN'T COPE?

_____

Guests

ADVICE FOR PARENTS (WE NEED IT)

_____

_____

_____

WISHES FOR THE MINI POOP MACHINE

_____

_____

_____

SLEEP (OR TRANQUILIZER) SUGGESTIONS

_____

YOU'RE KINDA GLAD IT'S NOT YOU, RIGHT?

_____

WILL YOU TAKE THIS CHILD IF WE CAN'T COPE?

_____

Guests

_____

ADVICE FOR PARENTS (WE NEED IT)

_____

_____

_____

WISHES FOR THE MINI POOP MACHINE

_____

_____

_____

SLEEP (OR TRANQUILIZER) SUGGESTIONS

_____

YOU'RE KINDA GLAD IT'S NOT YOU, RIGHT?

_____

WILL YOU TAKE THIS CHILD IF WE CAN'T COPE?

_____

Guests

ADVICE FOR PARENTS (WE NEED IT)

_____

_____

_____

WISHES FOR THE MINI POOP MACHINE

_____

_____

_____

SLEEP (OR TRANQUILIZER) SUGGESTIONS

_____

YOU'RE KINDA GLAD IT'S NOT YOU, RIGHT?

_____

WILL YOU TAKE THIS CHILD IF WE CAN'T COPE?

_____

Guests

ADVICE FOR PARENTS (WE NEED IT)

WISHES FOR THE MINI POOP MACHINE

SLEEP (OR TRANQUILIZER) SUGGESTIONS

YOU'RE KINDA GLAD IT'S NOT YOU, RIGHT?

WILL YOU TAKE THIS CHILD IF WE CAN'T COPE?

Guests

ADVICE FOR PARENTS (WE NEED IT)

_____

_____

_____

WISHES FOR THE MINI POOP MACHINE

_____

_____

_____

SLEEP (OR TRANQUILIZER) SUGGESTIONS

_____

YOU'RE KINDA GLAD IT'S NOT YOU, RIGHT?

_____

WILL YOU TAKE THIS CHILD IF WE CAN'T COPE?

_____

Guests

ADVICE FOR PARENTS (WE NEED IT)

WISHES FOR THE MINI POOP MACHINE

SLEEP (OR TRANQUILIZER) SUGGESTIONS

YOU'RE KINDA GLAD IT'S NOT YOU, RIGHT?

WILL YOU TAKE THIS CHILD IF WE CAN'T COPE?

Guests

ADVICE FOR PARENTS (WE NEED IT)

_____

_____

_____

WISHES FOR THE MINI POOP MACHINE

_____

_____

_____

SLEEP (OR TRANQUILIZER) SUGGESTIONS

_____

YOU'RE KINDA GLAD IT'S NOT YOU, RIGHT?

_____

WILL YOU TAKE THIS CHILD IF WE CAN'T COPE?

_____

Guests

_____

ADVICE FOR PARENTS (WE NEED IT)

_____

_____

_____

WISHES FOR THE MINI POOP MACHINE

_____

_____

_____

SLEEP (OR TRANQUILIZER) SUGGESTIONS

_____

YOU'RE KINDA GLAD IT'S NOT YOU, RIGHT?

_____

WILL YOU TAKE THIS CHILD IF WE CAN'T COPE?

_____

Guests

ADVICE FOR PARENTS (WE NEED IT)

_____

_____

_____

WISHES FOR THE MINI POOP MACHINE

_____

_____

_____

SLEEP (OR TRANQUILIZER) SUGGESTIONS

_____

YOU'RE KINDA GLAD IT'S NOT YOU, RIGHT?

_____

WILL YOU TAKE THIS CHILD IF WE CAN'T COPE?

_____

Guests

___

ADVICE FOR PARENTS (WE NEED IT)

___

___

___

WISHES FOR THE MINI POOP MACHINE

___

___

___

SLEEP (OR TRANQUILIZER) SUGGESTIONS

___

YOU'RE KINDA GLAD IT'S NOT YOU, RIGHT?

___

WILL YOU TAKE THIS CHILD IF WE CAN'T COPE?

___

Guests

ADVICE FOR PARENTS (WE NEED IT)

_____

_____

_____

WISHES FOR THE MINI POOP MACHINE

_____

_____

_____

SLEEP (OR TRANQUILIZER) SUGGESTIONS

_____

YOU'RE KINDA GLAD IT'S NOT YOU, RIGHT?

_____

WILL YOU TAKE THIS CHILD IF WE CAN'T COPE?

_____

Guests

_____

ADVICE FOR PARENTS (WE NEED IT)

_____

_____

_____

WISHES FOR THE MINI POOP MACHINE

_____

_____

_____

SLEEP (OR TRANQUILIZER) SUGGESTIONS

_____

YOU'RE KINDA GLAD IT'S NOT YOU, RIGHT?

_____

WILL YOU TAKE THIS CHILD IF WE CAN'T COPE?

_____

Guests

ADVICE FOR PARENTS (WE NEED IT)

_____

_____

_____

WISHES FOR THE MINI POOP MACHINE

_____

_____

_____

SLEEP (OR TRANQUILIZER) SUGGESTIONS

_____

YOU'RE KINDA GLAD IT'S NOT YOU, RIGHT?

_____

WILL YOU TAKE THIS CHILD IF WE CAN'T COPE?

_____

Guests

_____

ADVICE FOR PARENTS (WE NEED IT)

_____

_____

_____

WISHES FOR THE MINI POOP MACHINE

_____

_____

_____

SLEEP (OR TRANQUILIZER) SUGGESTIONS

_____

YOU'RE KINDA GLAD IT'S NOT YOU, RIGHT?

_____

WILL YOU TAKE THIS CHILD IF WE CAN'T COPE?

_____

Guests

ADVICE FOR PARENTS (WE NEED IT)

WISHES FOR THE MINI POOP MACHINE

SLEEP (OR TRANQUILIZER) SUGGESTIONS

YOU'RE KINDA GLAD IT'S NOT YOU, RIGHT?

WILL YOU TAKE THIS CHILD IF WE CAN'T COPE?

Guests

_____

ADVICE FOR PARENTS (WE NEED IT)

_____

_____

_____

WISHES FOR THE MINI POOP MACHINE

_____

_____

_____

SLEEP (OR TRANQUILIZER) SUGGESTIONS

_____

YOU'RE KINDA GLAD IT'S NOT YOU, RIGHT?

_____

WILL YOU TAKE THIS CHILD IF WE CAN'T COPE?

_____

Guests

ADVICE FOR PARENTS (WE NEED IT)

_____

_____

_____

WISHES FOR THE MINI POOP MACHINE

_____

_____

_____

SLEEP (OR TRANQUILIZER) SUGGESTIONS

_____

YOU'RE KINDA GLAD IT'S NOT YOU, RIGHT?

_____

WILL YOU TAKE THIS CHILD IF WE CAN'T COPE?

_____

Guests

ADVICE FOR PARENTS (WE NEED IT)

WISHES FOR THE MINI POOP MACHINE

SLEEP (OR TRANQUILIZER) SUGGESTIONS

YOU'RE KINDA GLAD IT'S NOT YOU, RIGHT?

WILL YOU TAKE THIS CHILD IF WE CAN'T COPE?

Guests

ADVICE FOR PARENTS (WE NEED IT)

_____

_____

_____

WISHES FOR THE MINI POOP MACHINE

_____

_____

_____

SLEEP (OR TRANQUILIZER) SUGGESTIONS

_____

YOU'RE KINDA GLAD IT'S NOT YOU, RIGHT?

_____

WILL YOU TAKE THIS CHILD IF WE CAN'T COPE?

_____

Guests

_____

ADVICE FOR PARENTS (WE NEED IT)

_____

_____

_____

WISHES FOR THE MINI POOP MACHINE

_____

_____

_____

SLEEP (OR TRANQUILIZER) SUGGESTIONS

_____

YOU'RE KINDA GLAD IT'S NOT YOU, RIGHT?

_____

WILL YOU TAKE THIS CHILD IF WE CAN'T COPE?

_____

Guests

_____

ADVICE FOR PARENTS (WE NEED IT)

_____

_____

_____

WISHES FOR THE MINI POOP MACHINE

_____

_____

_____

SLEEP (OR TRANQUILIZER) SUGGESTIONS

_____

YOU'RE KINDA GLAD IT'S NOT YOU, RIGHT?

_____

WILL YOU TAKE THIS CHILD IF WE CAN'T COPE?

_____

Guests

_____

ADVICE FOR PARENTS (WE NEED IT)

_____

_____

_____

WISHES FOR THE MINI POOP MACHINE

_____

_____

_____

SLEEP (OR TRANQUILIZER) SUGGESTIONS

_____

YOU'RE KINDA GLAD IT'S NOT YOU, RIGHT?

_____

WILL YOU TAKE THIS CHILD IF WE CAN'T COPE?

_____

Guests

ADVICE FOR PARENTS (WE NEED IT)

_____

_____

_____

WISHES FOR THE MINI POOP MACHINE

_____

_____

_____

SLEEP (OR TRANQUILIZER) SUGGESTIONS

_____

YOU'RE KINDA GLAD IT'S NOT YOU, RIGHT?

_____

WILL YOU TAKE THIS CHILD IF WE CAN'T COPE?

_____

Guests

_____

ADVICE FOR PARENTS (WE NEED IT)

_____

_____

_____

WISHES FOR THE MINI POOP MACHINE

_____

_____

SLEEP (OR TRANQUILIZER) SUGGESTIONS

_____

YOU'RE KINDA GLAD IT'S NOT YOU, RIGHT?

_____

WILL YOU TAKE THIS CHILD IF WE CAN'T COPE?

_____

Guests

ADVICE FOR PARENTS (WE NEED IT)

WISHES FOR THE MINI POOP MACHINE

SLEEP (OR TRANQUILIZER) SUGGESTIONS

YOU'RE KINDA GLAD IT'S NOT YOU, RIGHT?

WILL YOU TAKE THIS CHILD IF WE CAN'T COPE?

Guests

_____

ADVICE FOR PARENTS (WE NEED IT)

_____

_____

_____

WISHES FOR THE MINI POOP MACHINE

_____

_____

_____

SLEEP (OR TRANQUILIZER) SUGGESTIONS

_____

YOU'RE KINDA GLAD IT'S NOT YOU, RIGHT?

_____

WILL YOU TAKE THIS CHILD IF WE CAN'T COPE?

_____

Guests

ADVICE FOR PARENTS (WE NEED IT)

_____

_____

_____

WISHES FOR THE MINI POOP MACHINE

_____

_____

_____

SLEEP (OR TRANQUILIZER) SUGGESTIONS

_____

YOU'RE KINDA GLAD IT'S NOT YOU, RIGHT?

_____

WILL YOU TAKE THIS CHILD IF WE CAN'T COPE?

_____

Guests

_____

ADVICE FOR PARENTS (WE NEED IT)

_____

_____

_____

WISHES FOR THE MINI POOP MACHINE

_____

_____

_____

SLEEP (OR TRANQUILIZER) SUGGESTIONS

_____

YOU'RE KINDA GLAD IT'S NOT YOU, RIGHT?

_____

WILL YOU TAKE THIS CHILD IF WE CAN'T COPE?

_____

Guests

___

ADVICE FOR PARENTS (WE NEED IT)

___

___

___

WISHES FOR THE MINI POOP MACHINE

___

___

___

SLEEP (OR TRANQUILIZER) SUGGESTIONS

___

YOU'RE KINDA GLAD IT'S NOT YOU, RIGHT?

___

WILL YOU TAKE THIS CHILD IF WE CAN'T COPE?

___

Guests

ADVICE FOR PARENTS (WE NEED IT)

_____

_____

_____

WISHES FOR THE MINI POOP MACHINE

_____

_____

_____

SLEEP (OR TRANQUILIZER) SUGGESTIONS

_____

YOU'RE KINDA GLAD IT'S NOT YOU, RIGHT?

_____

WILL YOU TAKE THIS CHILD IF WE CAN'T COPE?

_____

Guests

ADVICE FOR PARENTS (WE NEED IT)

WISHES FOR THE MINI POOP MACHINE

SLEEP (OR TRANQUILIZER) SUGGESTIONS

YOU'RE KINDA GLAD IT'S NOT YOU, RIGHT?

WILL YOU TAKE THIS CHILD IF WE CAN'T COPE?

Guests

_____

ADVICE FOR PARENTS (WE NEED IT)

_____

_____

_____

WISHES FOR THE MINI POOP MACHINE

_____

_____

_____

SLEEP (OR TRANQUILIZER) SUGGESTIONS

_____

YOU'RE KINDA GLAD IT'S NOT YOU, RIGHT?

_____

WILL YOU TAKE THIS CHILD IF WE CAN'T COPE?

_____

Guests

ADVICE FOR PARENTS (WE NEED IT)

_____

_____

_____

WISHES FOR THE MINI POOP MACHINE

_____

_____

_____

SLEEP (OR TRANQUILIZER) SUGGESTIONS

_____

YOU'RE KINDA GLAD IT'S NOT YOU, RIGHT?

_____

WILL YOU TAKE THIS CHILD IF WE CAN'T COPE?

_____

Guests

_____

ADVICE FOR PARENTS (WE NEED IT)

_____

_____

_____

WISHES FOR THE MINI POOP MACHINE

_____

_____

_____

SLEEP (OR TRANQUILIZER) SUGGESTIONS

_____

YOU'RE KINDA GLAD IT'S NOT YOU, RIGHT?

_____

WILL YOU TAKE THIS CHILD IF WE CAN'T COPE?

_____

Guests

ADVICE FOR PARENTS (WE NEED IT)

_____

_____

_____

WISHES FOR THE MINI POOP MACHINE

_____

_____

_____

SLEEP (OR TRANQUILIZER) SUGGESTIONS

_____

YOU'RE KINDA GLAD IT'S NOT YOU, RIGHT?

_____

WILL YOU TAKE THIS CHILD IF WE CAN'T COPE?

_____

Guests

_____

ADVICE FOR PARENTS (WE NEED IT)

_____

_____

_____

WISHES FOR THE MINI POOP MACHINE

_____

_____

_____

SLEEP (OR TRANQUILIZER) SUGGESTIONS

_____

YOU'RE KINDA GLAD IT'S NOT YOU, RIGHT?

_____

WILL YOU TAKE THIS CHILD IF WE CAN'T COPE?

_____

Guests

ADVICE FOR PARENTS (WE NEED IT)

_____

_____

_____

WISHES FOR THE MINI POOP MACHINE

_____

_____

_____

SLEEP (OR TRANQUILIZER) SUGGESTIONS

_____

YOU'RE KINDA GLAD IT'S NOT YOU, RIGHT?

_____

WILL YOU TAKE THIS CHILD IF WE CAN'T COPE?

_____

Guests

_____

ADVICE FOR PARENTS (WE NEED IT)

_____

_____

_____

WISHES FOR THE MINI POOP MACHINE

_____

_____

_____

SLEEP (OR TRANQUILIZER) SUGGESTIONS

_____

YOU'RE KINDA GLAD IT'S NOT YOU, RIGHT?

_____

WILL YOU TAKE THIS CHILD IF WE CAN'T COPE?

_____

Guests

ADVICE FOR PARENTS (WE NEED IT)

_____

_____

_____

WISHES FOR THE MINI POOP MACHINE

_____

_____

_____

SLEEP (OR TRANQUILIZER) SUGGESTIONS

_____

YOU'RE KINDA GLAD IT'S NOT YOU, RIGHT?

_____

WILL YOU TAKE THIS CHILD IF WE CAN'T COPE?

_____

Guests

_____

ADVICE FOR PARENTS (WE NEED IT)

_____

_____

_____

WISHES FOR THE MINI POOP MACHINE

_____

_____

_____

SLEEP (OR TRANQUILIZER) SUGGESTIONS

_____

YOU'RE KINDA GLAD IT'S NOT YOU, RIGHT?

_____

WILL YOU TAKE THIS CHILD IF WE CAN'T COPE?

_____

Guests

ADVICE FOR PARENTS (WE NEED IT)

_____

_____

_____

WISHES FOR THE MINI POOP MACHINE

_____

_____

_____

SLEEP (OR TRANQUILIZER) SUGGESTIONS

_____

YOU'RE KINDA GLAD IT'S NOT YOU, RIGHT?

_____

WILL YOU TAKE THIS CHILD IF WE CAN'T COPE?

_____

Guests

_____

ADVICE FOR PARENTS (WE NEED IT)

_____

_____

_____

WISHES FOR THE MINI POOP MACHINE

_____

_____

_____

SLEEP (OR TRANQUILIZER) SUGGESTIONS

_____

YOU'RE KINDA GLAD IT'S NOT YOU, RIGHT?

_____

WILL YOU TAKE THIS CHILD IF WE CAN'T COPE?

_____

Guests

ADVICE FOR PARENTS (WE NEED IT)

WISHES FOR THE MINI POOP MACHINE

SLEEP (OR TRANQUILIZER) SUGGESTIONS

YOU'RE KINDA GLAD IT'S NOT YOU, RIGHT?

WILL YOU TAKE THIS CHILD IF WE CAN'T COPE?

Guests

_____

ADVICE FOR PARENTS (WE NEED IT)

_____

_____

_____

WISHES FOR THE MINI POOP MACHINE

_____

_____

_____

SLEEP (OR TRANQUILIZER) SUGGESTIONS

_____

YOU'RE KINDA GLAD IT'S NOT YOU, RIGHT?

_____

WILL YOU TAKE THIS CHILD IF WE CAN'T COPE?

_____

Guests

ADVICE FOR PARENTS (WE NEED IT)

_____

_____

_____

WISHES FOR THE MINI POOP MACHINE

_____

_____

_____

SLEEP (OR TRANQUILIZER) SUGGESTIONS

_____

YOU'RE KINDA GLAD IT'S NOT YOU, RIGHT?

_____

WILL YOU TAKE THIS CHILD IF WE CAN'T COPE?

_____

CPSIA information can be obtained
at www.ICGtesting.com
Printed in the USA
FSHW021949100320
68032FS

9 781913 357054